This tracking log belongs to:

IMPORTANT INFORMATION TO KNOW

Names of my diabetes medication(s) and dosage(s)

1. _____
2. _____
3. _____

Other Medication(s)

1. _____
2. _____
3. _____

My Doctor's Name: Phone #

_____   _____

Disclaimer: This information is intended for educational purposes only. It should not be interpreted as medical advice, diagnosis, or treatment and should not substitute for the professional advice of your physician or other qualified health care provider. If you have questions about a health condition, always seek the advice of your physician or other qualified health care provider.

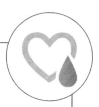

Congratulations on obtaining your Blood Sugar Tracking Log!

If you have been diagnosed with diabetes, tracking your blood sugar level is the first step in taking responsibility for your health. Tracking your blood sugar level helps you see the changes in your blood sugar and can allow you to better understand how physical activity, your food intake, and stress affect your blood sugar level. Tracking also helps you and your doctor understand how well your medication is working. Additionally, it's a way for you to track your progress in reaching your overall health and treatment goals.

According to The American Diabetes Association, a person with Type 2 diabetes should aim for a blood sugar level between 70 and 130 mg/dl before meals and less than 180 mg/dl one to two hours after a meal.

I hope you find this log helpful in tracking your blood sugar level and attaining your health goal!

VI Health & Wellness Coaching, LLC

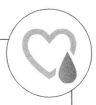

BLOOD SUGAR LEVEL CHART

Understanding the Numbers

Fasting

Normal for person without diabetes	70-99 mg/dl
Recommendation for someone with diabetes	80-130 mg/dl

Two Hours After Meals

Normal for person without diabetes	Less than 140 mg/dl
Recommendation for someone with diabetes	Less than 180 mg/dl

Hemoglobin A1C or HBA1C

Normal for person without diabetes	Less than 5.7%
Recommendation for someone with diabetes	Less than 7.0 %

Table 1. Data Source <u>American Diabetes Association</u>: The Big Picture: Checking Your Blood Pressure

HERE ARE TEN WAYS YOU CAN NATURALLY LOWER YOUR BLOOD SUGAR LEVEL:

- Exercise regularly.
- Control the amount of carbohydrates (starchy foods) you eat.
- Increase your fiber intake.
- Drink water and stay hydrated.
- Implement portion control when it comes to your meals and snacks.
- Choose foods with a low glycemic index (meaning foods that do not raise your blood sugar level).
- Control your stress level.
- Lose weight.
- Get high-quality sleep at night.
- Monitor and log your blood sugar level.

HOW TO COMPLETE YOUR BLOOD SUGAR LOG

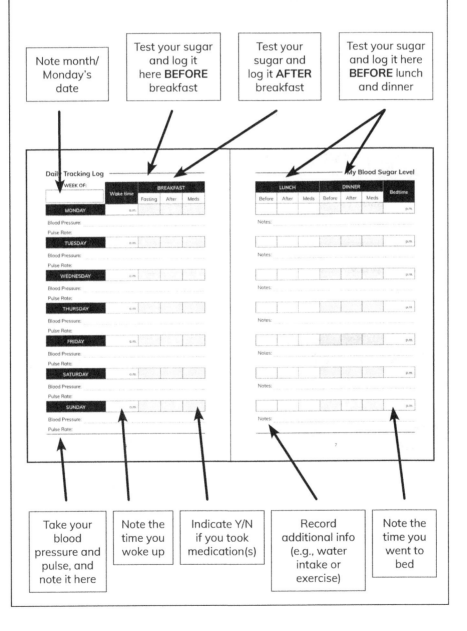

Daily Tracking Log

WEEK OF:	Wake time	BREAKFAST		
		Fasting	After	Meds
MONDAY	a.m.			

Blood Pressure: ....

Pulse Rate:

TUESDAY	a.m.			

Blood Pressure: ....

Pulse Rate:

WEDNESDAY	a.m.			

Blood Pressure: ....

Pulse Rate:

THURSDAY	a.m.			

Blood Pressure: ....

Pulse Rate:

FRIDAY	a.m.			

Blood Pressure: ....

Pulse Rate:

SATURDAY	a.m.			

Blood Pressure: ....

Pulse Rate:

SUNDAY	a.m.			

Blood Pressure: ....

Pulse Rate:

My Blood Sugar Level

LUNCH			DINNER			Bedtime
Before	After	Meds	Before	After	Meds	
						p.m.

Notes: ....

						p.m.

Notes: ....

						p.m.

Notes: ....

						p.m.

Notes: ....

						p.m.

Notes: ....

						p.m.

Notes: ....

						p.m.

Notes: ....

Daily Tracking Log

WEEK OF:	Wake time	BREAKFAST		
		Fasting	After	Meds
MONDAY	a.m.			

Blood Pressure: ....

Pulse Rate:

TUESDAY	a.m.			

Blood Pressure: ....

Pulse Rate:

WEDNESDAY	a.m.			

Blood Pressure: ....

Pulse Rate:

THURSDAY	a.m.			

Blood Pressure: ....

Pulse Rate:

FRIDAY	a.m.			

Blood Pressure: ....

Pulse Rate:

SATURDAY	a.m.			

Blood Pressure: ....

Pulse Rate:

SUNDAY	a.m.			

Blood Pressure: ....

Pulse Rate:

My Blood Sugar Level

LUNCH			DINNER			Bedtime
Before	After	Meds	Before	After	Meds	
						p.m.

Notes: ....

						p.m.

Notes: ....

						p.m.

Notes: ....

						p.m.

Notes: ....

						p.m.

Notes: ....

						p.m.

Notes: ....

						p.m.

Notes: ....

Daily Tracking Log

WEEK OF:	Wake time	BREAKFAST		
		Fasting	After	Meds
MONDAY	a.m.			

Blood Pressure: ....

Pulse Rate:

TUESDAY	a.m.			

Blood Pressure: ....

Pulse Rate:

WEDNESDAY	a.m.			

Blood Pressure: ....

Pulse Rate:

THURSDAY	a.m.			

Blood Pressure: ....

Pulse Rate:

FRIDAY	a.m.			

Blood Pressure: ....

Pulse Rate:

SATURDAY	a.m.			

Blood Pressure: ....

Pulse Rate:

SUNDAY	a.m.			

Blood Pressure: ....

Pulse Rate:

My Blood Sugar Level

LUNCH			DINNER			Bedtime
Before	After	Meds	Before	After	Meds	
						p.m.

Notes: ....

						p.m.

Notes: ....

						p.m.

Notes: ....

						p.m.

Notes: ....

						p.m.

Notes: ....

						p.m.

Notes: ....

						p.m.

Notes: ....

Daily Tracking Log

WEEK OF:	Wake time	BREAKFAST		
		Fasting	After	Meds
MONDAY	a.m.			

Blood Pressure: ....

Pulse Rate:

TUESDAY	a.m.			

Blood Pressure: ....

Pulse Rate:

WEDNESDAY	a.m.			

Blood Pressure: ....

Pulse Rate:

THURSDAY	a.m.			

Blood Pressure: ....

Pulse Rate:

FRIDAY	a.m.			

Blood Pressure: ....

Pulse Rate:

SATURDAY	a.m.			

Blood Pressure: ....

Pulse Rate:

SUNDAY	a.m.			

Blood Pressure: ....

Pulse Rate:

My Blood Sugar Level

LUNCH			DINNER			Bedtime
Before	After	Meds	Before	After	Meds	
						p.m.

Notes: ....

						p.m.

Notes: ....

						p.m.

Notes: ....

						p.m.

Notes: ....

						p.m.

Notes: ....

						p.m.

Notes: ....

						p.m.

Notes: ....

Daily Tracking Log

WEEK OF:	Wake time	BREAKFAST		
		Fasting	After	Meds
MONDAY	a.m.			

Blood Pressure: ....

Pulse Rate:

TUESDAY	a.m.			

Blood Pressure: ....

Pulse Rate:

WEDNESDAY	a.m.			

Blood Pressure: ....

Pulse Rate:

THURSDAY	a.m.			

Blood Pressure: ....

Pulse Rate:

FRIDAY	a.m.			

Blood Pressure: ....

Pulse Rate:

SATURDAY	a.m.			

Blood Pressure: ....

Pulse Rate:

SUNDAY	a.m.			

Blood Pressure: ....

Pulse Rate:

My Blood Sugar Level

LUNCH			DINNER			Bedtime
Before	After	Meds	Before	After	Meds	
						p.m.

Notes: ....

						p.m.

Notes: ....

						p.m.

Notes: ....

						p.m.

Notes: ....

						p.m.

Notes: ....

						p.m.

Notes: ....

						p.m.

Notes: ....

Daily Tracking Log

WEEK OF:	Wake time	BREAKFAST		
		Fasting	After	Meds
MONDAY	a.m.			

Blood Pressure: ....

Pulse Rate:

TUESDAY	a.m.			

Blood Pressure: ....

Pulse Rate:

WEDNESDAY	a.m.			

Blood Pressure: ....

Pulse Rate:

THURSDAY	a.m.			

Blood Pressure: ....

Pulse Rate:

FRIDAY	a.m.			

Blood Pressure: ....

Pulse Rate:

SATURDAY	a.m.			

Blood Pressure: ....

Pulse Rate:

SUNDAY	a.m.			

Blood Pressure: ....

Pulse Rate:

My Blood Sugar Level

LUNCH			DINNER			Bedtime
Before	After	Meds	Before	After	Meds	
						p.m.

Notes: ....

						p.m.

Notes: ....

						p.m.

Notes: ....

						p.m.

Notes: ....

						p.m.

Notes: ....

						p.m.

Notes: ....

						p.m.

Notes: ....

Daily Tracking Log

WEEK OF:	Wake time	BREAKFAST		
		Fasting	After	Meds
MONDAY	a.m.			

Blood Pressure: ....

Pulse Rate:

TUESDAY	a.m.			

Blood Pressure: ....

Pulse Rate:

WEDNESDAY	a.m.			

Blood Pressure: ....

Pulse Rate:

THURSDAY	a.m.			

Blood Pressure: ....

Pulse Rate:

FRIDAY	a.m.			

Blood Pressure: ....

Pulse Rate:

SATURDAY	a.m.			

Blood Pressure: ....

Pulse Rate:

SUNDAY	a.m.			

Blood Pressure: ....

Pulse Rate:

My Blood Sugar Level

LUNCH			DINNER			Bedtime
Before	After	Meds	Before	After	Meds	
						p.m.

Notes: ....

						p.m.

Notes: ....

						p.m.

Notes: ....

						p.m.

Notes: ....

						p.m.

Notes: ....

						p.m.

Notes: ....

						p.m.

Notes: ....

Daily Tracking Log

WEEK OF:	Wake time	BREAKFAST		
		Fasting	After	Meds
MONDAY	a.m.			

Blood Pressure: ....

Pulse Rate:

TUESDAY	a.m.			

Blood Pressure: ....

Pulse Rate:

WEDNESDAY	a.m.			

Blood Pressure: ....

Pulse Rate:

THURSDAY	a.m.			

Blood Pressure: ....

Pulse Rate:

FRIDAY	a.m.			

Blood Pressure: ....

Pulse Rate:

SATURDAY	a.m.			

Blood Pressure: ....

Pulse Rate:

SUNDAY	a.m.			

Blood Pressure: ....

Pulse Rate:

My Blood Sugar Level

LUNCH			DINNER			Bedtime
Before	After	Meds	Before	After	Meds	
						p.m.

Notes: ....

						p.m.

Notes: ....

						p.m.

Notes: ....

						p.m.

Notes: ....

						p.m.

Notes: ....

						p.m.

Notes: ....

						p.m.

Notes: ....

Daily Tracking Log

WEEK OF:	Wake time	BREAKFAST		
		Fasting	After	Meds
MONDAY	a.m.			

Blood Pressure: ....

Pulse Rate:

TUESDAY	a.m.			

Blood Pressure: ....

Pulse Rate:

WEDNESDAY	a.m.			

Blood Pressure: ....

Pulse Rate:

THURSDAY	a.m.			

Blood Pressure: ....

Pulse Rate:

FRIDAY	a.m.			

Blood Pressure: ....

Pulse Rate:

SATURDAY	a.m.			

Blood Pressure: ....

Pulse Rate:

SUNDAY	a.m.			

Blood Pressure: ....

Pulse Rate:

_____ **My Blood Sugar Level**

	LUNCH			DINNER			Bedtime
Before	After	Meds	Before	After	Meds		
							p.m.

Notes: ....

							p.m.

Notes: ....

							p.m.

Notes: ....

							p.m.

Notes: ....

							p.m.

Notes: ....

							p.m.

Notes: ....

							p.m.

Notes: ....

Daily Tracking Log

WEEK OF:	Wake time	BREAKFAST		
		Fasting	After	Meds
MONDAY	a.m.			

Blood Pressure: ....

Pulse Rate:

TUESDAY	a.m.			

Blood Pressure: ....

Pulse Rate:

WEDNESDAY	a.m.			

Blood Pressure: ....

Pulse Rate:

THURSDAY	a.m.			

Blood Pressure: ....

Pulse Rate:

FRIDAY	a.m.			

Blood Pressure: ....

Pulse Rate:

SATURDAY	a.m.			

Blood Pressure: ....

Pulse Rate:

SUNDAY	a.m.			

Blood Pressure: ....

Pulse Rate:

My Blood Sugar Level

LUNCH			DINNER			Bedtime
Before	After	Meds	Before	After	Meds	
						p.m.

Notes: ....

						p.m.

Notes: ....

						p.m.

Notes: ....

						p.m.

Notes: ....

						p.m.

Notes: ....

						p.m.

Notes: ....

						p.m.

Notes: ....

Daily Tracking Log

WEEK OF:	Wake time	BREAKFAST		
		Fasting	After	Meds
MONDAY	a.m.			

Blood Pressure: ....

Pulse Rate:

TUESDAY	a.m.			

Blood Pressure: ....

Pulse Rate:

WEDNESDAY	a.m.			

Blood Pressure: ....

Pulse Rate:

THURSDAY	a.m.			

Blood Pressure: ....

Pulse Rate:

FRIDAY	a.m.			

Blood Pressure: ....

Pulse Rate:

SATURDAY	a.m.			

Blood Pressure: ....

Pulse Rate:

SUNDAY	a.m.			

Blood Pressure: ....

Pulse Rate:

My Blood Sugar Level

LUNCH			DINNER			Bedtime
Before	After	Meds	Before	After	Meds	
						p.m.

Notes: ....

						p.m.

Notes: ....

						p.m.

Notes: ....

						p.m.

Notes: ....

						p.m.

Notes: ....

						p.m.

Notes: ....

						p.m.

Notes: ....

Daily Tracking Log

WEEK OF:	Wake time	BREAKFAST		
		Fasting	After	Meds
MONDAY	a.m.			

Blood Pressure: ....

Pulse Rate:

TUESDAY	a.m.			

Blood Pressure: ....

Pulse Rate:

WEDNESDAY	a.m.			

Blood Pressure: ....

Pulse Rate:

THURSDAY	a.m.			

Blood Pressure: ....

Pulse Rate:

FRIDAY	a.m.			

Blood Pressure: ....

Pulse Rate:

SATURDAY	a.m.			

Blood Pressure: ....

Pulse Rate:

SUNDAY	a.m.			

Blood Pressure: ....

Pulse Rate:

My Blood Sugar Level

LUNCH			DINNER			Bedtime
Before	After	Meds	Before	After	Meds	
						p.m.

Notes: ....

						p.m.

Notes: ....

						p.m.

Notes: ....

						p.m.

Notes: ....

						p.m.

Notes: ....

						p.m.

Notes: ....

						p.m.

Notes: ....

Daily Tracking Log

WEEK OF:	Wake time	BREAKFAST		
		Fasting	After	Meds
MONDAY	a.m.			

Blood Pressure: ....

Pulse Rate:

TUESDAY	a.m.			

Blood Pressure: ....

Pulse Rate:

WEDNESDAY	a.m.			

Blood Pressure: ....

Pulse Rate:

THURSDAY	a.m.			

Blood Pressure: ....

Pulse Rate:

FRIDAY	a.m.			

Blood Pressure: ....

Pulse Rate:

SATURDAY	a.m.			

Blood Pressure: ....

Pulse Rate:

SUNDAY	a.m.			

Blood Pressure: ....

Pulse Rate:

My Blood Sugar Level

LUNCH			DINNER			Bedtime
Before	After	Meds	Before	After	Meds	
						p.m.

Notes: ....

						p.m.

Notes: ....

						p.m.

Notes: ....

						p.m.

Notes: ....

						p.m.

Notes: ....

						p.m.

Notes: ....

						p.m.

Notes: ....

Daily Tracking Log

WEEK OF:	Wake time	BREAKFAST		
		Fasting	After	Meds
MONDAY	a.m.			

Blood Pressure: ....

Pulse Rate:

TUESDAY	a.m.			

Blood Pressure: ....

Pulse Rate:

WEDNESDAY	a.m.			

Blood Pressure: ....

Pulse Rate:

THURSDAY	a.m.			

Blood Pressure: ....

Pulse Rate:

FRIDAY	a.m.			

Blood Pressure: ....

Pulse Rate:

SATURDAY	a.m.			

Blood Pressure: ....

Pulse Rate:

SUNDAY	a.m.			

Blood Pressure: ....

Pulse Rate:

My Blood Sugar Level

LUNCH			DINNER			Bedtime
Before	After	Meds	Before	After	Meds	
						p.m.

Notes: ....

						p.m.

Notes: ....

						p.m.

Notes: ....

						p.m.

Notes: ....

						p.m.

Notes: ....

						p.m.

Notes: ....

						p.m.

Notes: ....

Daily Tracking Log

WEEK OF:	Wake time	BREAKFAST		
		Fasting	After	Meds
MONDAY	a.m.			

Blood Pressure: ....

Pulse Rate:

TUESDAY	a.m.			

Blood Pressure: ....

Pulse Rate:

WEDNESDAY	a.m.			

Blood Pressure: ....

Pulse Rate:

THURSDAY	a.m.			

Blood Pressure: ....

Pulse Rate:

FRIDAY	a.m.			

Blood Pressure: ....

Pulse Rate:

SATURDAY	a.m.			

Blood Pressure: ....

Pulse Rate:

SUNDAY	a.m.			

Blood Pressure: ....

Pulse Rate:

My Blood Sugar Level

LUNCH			DINNER			Bedtime
Before	After	Meds	Before	After	Meds	
						p.m.

Notes: ....

						p.m.

Notes: ....

						p.m.

Notes: ....

						p.m.

Notes: ....

						p.m.

Notes: ....

						p.m.

Notes: ....

						p.m.

Notes: ....

Daily Tracking Log

WEEK OF:	Wake time	BREAKFAST		
		Fasting	After	Meds
MONDAY	a.m.			

Blood Pressure: ....

Pulse Rate:

TUESDAY	a.m.			

Blood Pressure: ....

Pulse Rate:

WEDNESDAY	a.m.			

Blood Pressure: ....

Pulse Rate:

THURSDAY	a.m.			

Blood Pressure: ....

Pulse Rate:

FRIDAY	a.m.			

Blood Pressure: ....

Pulse Rate:

SATURDAY	a.m.			

Blood Pressure: ....

Pulse Rate:

SUNDAY	a.m.			

Blood Pressure: ....

Pulse Rate:

My Blood Sugar Level

LUNCH			DINNER			Bedtime
Before	After	Meds	Before	After	Meds	
						p.m.

Notes: ....

						p.m.

Notes: ....

						p.m.

Notes: ....

						p.m.

Notes: ....

						p.m.

Notes: ....

						p.m.

Notes: ....

						p.m.

Notes: ....

Daily Tracking Log

WEEK OF:	Wake time	BREAKFAST		
		Fasting	After	Meds
MONDAY	a.m.			

Blood Pressure: ....

Pulse Rate:

TUESDAY	a.m.			

Blood Pressure: ....

Pulse Rate:

WEDNESDAY	a.m.			

Blood Pressure: ....

Pulse Rate:

THURSDAY	a.m.			

Blood Pressure: ....

Pulse Rate:

FRIDAY	a.m.			

Blood Pressure: ....

Pulse Rate:

SATURDAY	a.m.			

Blood Pressure: ....

Pulse Rate:

SUNDAY	a.m.			

Blood Pressure: ....

Pulse Rate:

My Blood Sugar Level

LUNCH			DINNER			Bedtime
Before	After	Meds	Before	After	Meds	
						p.m.

Notes: ....

						p.m.

Notes: ....

						p.m.

Notes: ....

						p.m.

Notes: ....

						p.m.

Notes: ....

						p.m.

Notes: ....

						p.m.

Notes: ....

Daily Tracking Log

WEEK OF:	Wake time	BREAKFAST		
		Fasting	After	Meds
MONDAY	a.m.			

Blood Pressure: ....

Pulse Rate:

TUESDAY	a.m.			

Blood Pressure: ....

Pulse Rate:

WEDNESDAY	a.m.			

Blood Pressure: ....

Pulse Rate:

THURSDAY	a.m.			

Blood Pressure: ....

Pulse Rate:

FRIDAY	a.m.			

Blood Pressure: ....

Pulse Rate:

SATURDAY	a.m.			

Blood Pressure: ....

Pulse Rate:

SUNDAY	a.m.			

Blood Pressure: ....

Pulse Rate:

My Blood Sugar Level

LUNCH			DINNER			Bedtime
Before	After	Meds	Before	After	Meds	
						p.m.

Notes: ....

						p.m.

Notes: ....

						p.m.

Notes: ....

						p.m.

Notes: ....

						p.m.

Notes: ....

						p.m.

Notes: ....

						p.m.

Notes: ....

Daily Tracking Log

WEEK OF:	Wake time	BREAKFAST		
		Fasting	After	Meds
MONDAY	a.m.			

Blood Pressure: ....

Pulse Rate:

TUESDAY	a.m.			

Blood Pressure: ....

Pulse Rate:

WEDNESDAY	a.m.			

Blood Pressure: ....

Pulse Rate:

THURSDAY	a.m.			

Blood Pressure: ....

Pulse Rate:

FRIDAY	a.m.			

Blood Pressure: ....

Pulse Rate:

SATURDAY	a.m.			

Blood Pressure: ....

Pulse Rate:

SUNDAY	a.m.			

Blood Pressure: ....

Pulse Rate:

My Blood Sugar Level

LUNCH			DINNER			Bedtime
Before	After	Meds	Before	After	Meds	
						p.m.

Notes: ....

						p.m.

Notes: ....

						p.m.

Notes: ....

						p.m.

Notes: ....

						p.m.

Notes: ....

						p.m.

Notes: ....

						p.m.

Notes: ....

Daily Tracking Log

WEEK OF:	Wake time	BREAKFAST		
		Fasting	After	Meds
MONDAY	a.m.			

Blood Pressure: ....

Pulse Rate:

TUESDAY	a.m.			

Blood Pressure: ....

Pulse Rate:

WEDNESDAY	a.m.			

Blood Pressure: ....

Pulse Rate:

THURSDAY	a.m.			

Blood Pressure: ....

Pulse Rate:

FRIDAY	a.m.			

Blood Pressure: ....

Pulse Rate:

SATURDAY	a.m.			

Blood Pressure: ....

Pulse Rate:

SUNDAY	a.m.			

Blood Pressure: ....

Pulse Rate:

My Blood Sugar Level

LUNCH			DINNER			Bedtime
Before	After	Meds	Before	After	Meds	
						p.m.

Notes: ....

						p.m.

Notes: ....

						p.m.

Notes: ....

						p.m.

Notes: ....

						p.m.

Notes: ....

						p.m.

Notes: ....

						p.m.

Notes: ....

Daily Tracking Log

WEEK OF:	Wake time	BREAKFAST		
		Fasting	After	Meds
MONDAY	a.m.			

Blood Pressure:

Pulse Rate:

TUESDAY	a.m.			

Blood Pressure:

Pulse Rate:

WEDNESDAY	a.m.			

Blood Pressure:

Pulse Rate:

THURSDAY	a.m.			

Blood Pressure:

Pulse Rate:

FRIDAY	a.m.			

Blood Pressure:

Pulse Rate:

SATURDAY	a.m.			

Blood Pressure:

Pulse Rate:

SUNDAY	a.m.			

Blood Pressure:

Pulse Rate:

My Blood Sugar Level

LUNCH			DINNER			Bedtime
Before	After	Meds	Before	After	Meds	
						p.m.

Notes: ....

						p.m.

Notes: ....

						p.m.

Notes: ....

						p.m.

Notes: ....

						p.m.

Notes: ....

						p.m.

Notes: ....

						p.m.

Notes: ....

Daily Tracking Log

WEEK OF:	Wake time	BREAKFAST		
		Fasting	After	Meds
MONDAY	a.m.			

Blood Pressure: ....

Pulse Rate:

TUESDAY	a.m.			

Blood Pressure: ....

Pulse Rate:

WEDNESDAY	a.m.			

Blood Pressure: ....

Pulse Rate:

THURSDAY	a.m.			

Blood Pressure: ....

Pulse Rate:

FRIDAY	a.m.			

Blood Pressure: ....

Pulse Rate:

SATURDAY	a.m.			

Blood Pressure: ....

Pulse Rate:

SUNDAY	a.m.			

Blood Pressure: ....

Pulse Rate:

My Blood Sugar Level

LUNCH			DINNER			Bedtime
Before	After	Meds	Before	After	Meds	
						p.m.

Notes: ....

						p.m.

Notes: ....

						p.m.

Notes: ....

						p.m.

Notes: ....

						p.m.

Notes: ....

						p.m.

Notes: ....

						p.m.

Notes: ....

Daily Tracking Log

WEEK OF:	Wake time	BREAKFAST		
		Fasting	After	Meds
MONDAY	a.m.			

Blood Pressure: ....

Pulse Rate:

TUESDAY	a.m.			

Blood Pressure: ....

Pulse Rate:

WEDNESDAY	a.m.			

Blood Pressure: ....

Pulse Rate:

THURSDAY	a.m.			

Blood Pressure: ....

Pulse Rate:

FRIDAY	a.m.			

Blood Pressure: ....

Pulse Rate:

SATURDAY	a.m.			

Blood Pressure: ....

Pulse Rate:

SUNDAY	a.m.			

Blood Pressure: ....

Pulse Rate:

My Blood Sugar Level

LUNCH			DINNER			Bedtime
Before	After	Meds	Before	After	Meds	
						p.m.

Notes: ....

						p.m.

Notes: ....

						p.m.

Notes: ....

						p.m.

Notes: ....

						p.m.

Notes: ....

						p.m.

Notes: ....

						p.m.

Notes: ....

Daily Tracking Log

WEEK OF:	Wake time	BREAKFAST		
		Fasting	After	Meds
MONDAY	a.m.			

Blood Pressure: ....

Pulse Rate:

TUESDAY	a.m.			

Blood Pressure: ....

Pulse Rate:

WEDNESDAY	a.m.			

Blood Pressure: ....

Pulse Rate:

THURSDAY	a.m.			

Blood Pressure: ....

Pulse Rate:

FRIDAY	a.m.			

Blood Pressure: ....

Pulse Rate:

SATURDAY	a.m.			

Blood Pressure: ....

Pulse Rate:

SUNDAY	a.m.			

Blood Pressure: ....

Pulse Rate:

My Blood Sugar Level

LUNCH			DINNER			Bedtime
Before	After	Meds	Before	After	Meds	
						p.m.

Notes: ....

						p.m.

Notes: ....

						p.m.

Notes: ....

						p.m.

Notes: ....

						p.m.

Notes: ....

						p.m.

Notes: ....

						p.m.

Notes: ....

Daily Tracking Log

WEEK OF:	Wake time	BREAKFAST		
		Fasting	After	Meds
MONDAY	a.m.			

Blood Pressure: ....

Pulse Rate:

TUESDAY	a.m.			

Blood Pressure: ....

Pulse Rate:

WEDNESDAY	a.m.			

Blood Pressure: ....

Pulse Rate:

THURSDAY	a.m.			

Blood Pressure: ....

Pulse Rate:

FRIDAY	a.m.			

Blood Pressure: ....

Pulse Rate:

SATURDAY	a.m.			

Blood Pressure: ....

Pulse Rate:

SUNDAY	a.m.			

Blood Pressure: ....

Pulse Rate:

My Blood Sugar Level

LUNCH			DINNER			Bedtime
Before	After	Meds	Before	After	Meds	
						p.m.

Notes: ....

						p.m.

Notes: ....

						p.m.

Notes: ....

						p.m.

Notes: ....

						p.m.

Notes: ....

						p.m.

Notes: ....

						p.m.

Notes: ....

Daily Tracking Log

WEEK OF:	Wake time	BREAKFAST		
		Fasting	After	Meds
MONDAY	a.m.			

Blood Pressure: ....

Pulse Rate:

TUESDAY	a.m.			

Blood Pressure: ....

Pulse Rate:

WEDNESDAY	a.m.			

Blood Pressure: ....

Pulse Rate:

THURSDAY	a.m.			

Blood Pressure: ....

Pulse Rate:

FRIDAY	a.m.			

Blood Pressure: ....

Pulse Rate:

SATURDAY	a.m.			

Blood Pressure: ....

Pulse Rate:

SUNDAY	a.m.			

Blood Pressure: ....

Pulse Rate:

My Blood Sugar Level

LUNCH			DINNER			Bedtime
Before	After	Meds	Before	After	Meds	
						p.m.

Notes: ....

						p.m.

Notes: ....

						p.m.

Notes: ....

						p.m.

Notes: ....

						p.m.

Notes: ....

						p.m.

Notes: ....

						p.m.

Notes: ....

Daily Tracking Log

WEEK OF:	Wake time	BREAKFAST		
		Fasting	After	Meds
MONDAY	a.m.			

Blood Pressure: ....

Pulse Rate:

TUESDAY	a.m.			

Blood Pressure: ....

Pulse Rate:

WEDNESDAY	a.m.			

Blood Pressure: ....

Pulse Rate:

THURSDAY	a.m.			

Blood Pressure: ....

Pulse Rate:

FRIDAY	a.m.			

Blood Pressure: ....

Pulse Rate:

SATURDAY	a.m.			

Blood Pressure: ....

Pulse Rate:

SUNDAY	a.m.			

Blood Pressure: ....

Pulse Rate:

My Blood Sugar Level

LUNCH			DINNER			Bedtime
Before	After	Meds	Before	After	Meds	
						p.m.

Notes: ....

| | | | | | | p.m. |

Notes: ....

| | | | | | | p.m. |

Notes: ....

| | | | | | | p.m. |

Notes: ....

| | | | | | | p.m. |

Notes: ....

| | | | | | | p.m. |

Notes: ....

| | | | | | | p.m. |

Notes: ....

Daily Tracking Log

WEEK OF:	Wake time	BREAKFAST		
		Fasting	After	Meds
MONDAY	a.m.			

Blood Pressure: ....

Pulse Rate:

TUESDAY	a.m.			

Blood Pressure: ....

Pulse Rate:

WEDNESDAY	a.m.			

Blood Pressure: ....

Pulse Rate:

THURSDAY	a.m.			

Blood Pressure: ....

Pulse Rate:

FRIDAY	a.m.			

Blood Pressure: ....

Pulse Rate:

SATURDAY	a.m.			

Blood Pressure: ....

Pulse Rate:

SUNDAY	a.m.			

Blood Pressure: ....

Pulse Rate:

My Blood Sugar Level

LUNCH			DINNER			Bedtime
Before	After	Meds	Before	After	Meds	
						p.m.

Notes: ....

						p.m.

Notes: ....

						p.m.

Notes: ....

						p.m.

Notes: ....

						p.m.

Notes: ....

						p.m.

Notes: ....

						p.m.

Notes: ....

Daily Tracking Log

WEEK OF:	Wake time	BREAKFAST		
		Fasting	After	Meds
MONDAY	a.m.			

Blood Pressure: ....

Pulse Rate:

TUESDAY	a.m.			

Blood Pressure: ....

Pulse Rate:

WEDNESDAY	a.m.			

Blood Pressure: ....

Pulse Rate:

THURSDAY	a.m.			

Blood Pressure: ....

Pulse Rate:

FRIDAY	a.m.			

Blood Pressure: ....

Pulse Rate:

SATURDAY	a.m.			

Blood Pressure: ....

Pulse Rate:

SUNDAY	a.m.			

Blood Pressure: ....

Pulse Rate:

My Blood Sugar Level

	LUNCH			DINNER			Bedtime
Before	After	Meds	Before	After	Meds		
							p.m.

Notes: ....

							p.m.

Notes: ....

							p.m.

Notes: ....

							p.m.

Notes: ....

							p.m.

Notes: ....

							p.m.

Notes: ....

							p.m.

Notes: ....

Daily Tracking Log

WEEK OF:	Wake time	BREAKFAST		
		Fasting	After	Meds
MONDAY	a.m.			

Blood Pressure: ....

Pulse Rate:

TUESDAY	a.m.			

Blood Pressure: ....

Pulse Rate:

WEDNESDAY	a.m.			

Blood Pressure: ....

Pulse Rate:

THURSDAY	a.m.			

Blood Pressure: ....

Pulse Rate:

FRIDAY	a.m.			

Blood Pressure: ....

Pulse Rate:

SATURDAY	a.m.			

Blood Pressure: ....

Pulse Rate:

SUNDAY	a.m.			

Blood Pressure: ....

Pulse Rate:

My Blood Sugar Level

LUNCH			DINNER			Bedtime
Before	After	Meds	Before	After	Meds	
						p.m.

Notes: ....

						p.m.

Notes: ....

						p.m.

Notes: ....

						p.m.

Notes: ....

						p.m.

Notes: ....

						p.m.

Notes: ....

						p.m.

Notes: ....

Daily Tracking Log

WEEK OF:	Wake time	BREAKFAST		
		Fasting	After	Meds
MONDAY	a.m.			

Blood Pressure: ....

Pulse Rate:

TUESDAY	a.m.			

Blood Pressure: ....

Pulse Rate:

WEDNESDAY	a.m.			

Blood Pressure: ....

Pulse Rate:

THURSDAY	a.m.			

Blood Pressure: ....

Pulse Rate:

FRIDAY	a.m.			

Blood Pressure: ....

Pulse Rate:

SATURDAY	a.m.			

Blood Pressure: ....

Pulse Rate:

SUNDAY	a.m.			

Blood Pressure: ....

Pulse Rate:

My Blood Sugar Level

LUNCH			DINNER			Bedtime
Before	After	Meds	Before	After	Meds	
						p.m.

Notes: ....

						p.m.

Notes: ....

						p.m.

Notes: ....

						p.m.

Notes: ....

						p.m.

Notes: ....

						p.m.

Notes: ....

						p.m.

Notes: ....

Daily Tracking Log

WEEK OF:	Wake time	BREAKFAST		
		Fasting	After	Meds
MONDAY	a.m.			

Blood Pressure: ......

Pulse Rate:

TUESDAY	a.m.			

Blood Pressure: ......

Pulse Rate:

WEDNESDAY	a.m.			

Blood Pressure: ......

Pulse Rate:

THURSDAY	a.m.			

Blood Pressure: ......

Pulse Rate:

FRIDAY	a.m.			

Blood Pressure: ......

Pulse Rate:

SATURDAY	a.m.			

Blood Pressure: ......

Pulse Rate:

SUNDAY	a.m.			

Blood Pressure: ......

Pulse Rate:

My Blood Sugar Level

LUNCH			DINNER			Bedtime
Before	After	Meds	Before	After	Meds	
						p.m.

Notes: ....

						p.m.

Notes: ....

						p.m.

Notes: ....

						p.m.

Notes: ....

						p.m.

Notes: ....

						p.m.

Notes: ....

						p.m.

Notes: ....

Daily Tracking Log

WEEK OF:	Wake time	BREAKFAST		
		Fasting	After	Meds
MONDAY	a.m.			

Blood Pressure: ....

Pulse Rate:

TUESDAY	a.m.			

Blood Pressure: ....

Pulse Rate:

WEDNESDAY	a.m.			

Blood Pressure: ....

Pulse Rate:

THURSDAY	a.m.			

Blood Pressure: ....

Pulse Rate:

FRIDAY	a.m.			

Blood Pressure: ....

Pulse Rate:

SATURDAY	a.m.			

Blood Pressure: ....

Pulse Rate:

SUNDAY	a.m.			

Blood Pressure: ....

Pulse Rate:

My Blood Sugar Level

LUNCH			DINNER			Bedtime
Before	After	Meds	Before	After	Meds	
						p.m.

Notes: ....

						p.m.

Notes: ....

						p.m.

Notes: ....

						p.m.

Notes: ....

						p.m.

Notes: ....

						p.m.

Notes: ....

						p.m.

Notes: ....

Daily Tracking Log

WEEK OF:	Wake time	BREAKFAST		
		Fasting	After	Meds
MONDAY	a.m.			

Blood Pressure: ....

Pulse Rate:

TUESDAY	a.m.			

Blood Pressure: ....

Pulse Rate:

WEDNESDAY	a.m.			

Blood Pressure: ....

Pulse Rate:

THURSDAY	a.m.			

Blood Pressure: ....

Pulse Rate:

FRIDAY	a.m.			

Blood Pressure: ....

Pulse Rate:

SATURDAY	a.m.			

Blood Pressure: ....

Pulse Rate:

SUNDAY	a.m.			

Blood Pressure: ....

Pulse Rate:

My Blood Sugar Level

LUNCH			DINNER			Bedtime
Before	After	Meds	Before	After	Meds	
						p.m.

Notes: ....

						p.m.

Notes: ....

						p.m.

Notes: ....

						p.m.

Notes: ....

						p.m.

Notes: ....

						p.m.

Notes: ....

						p.m.

Notes: ....

Daily Tracking Log

WEEK OF:	Wake time	BREAKFAST		
		Fasting	After	Meds
MONDAY	a.m.			

Blood Pressure: ....

Pulse Rate:

TUESDAY	a.m.			

Blood Pressure: ....

Pulse Rate:

WEDNESDAY	a.m.			

Blood Pressure: ....

Pulse Rate:

THURSDAY	a.m.			

Blood Pressure: ....

Pulse Rate:

FRIDAY	a.m.			

Blood Pressure: ....

Pulse Rate:

SATURDAY	a.m.			

Blood Pressure: ....

Pulse Rate:

SUNDAY	a.m.			

Blood Pressure: ....

Pulse Rate:

My Blood Sugar Level

	LUNCH			DINNER			Bedtime
Before	After	Meds	Before	After	Meds		
							p.m.

Notes: ....

							p.m.

Notes: ....

							p.m.

Notes: ....

							p.m.

Notes: ....

							p.m.

Notes: ....

							p.m.

Notes: ....

							p.m.

Notes: ....

Daily Tracking Log

WEEK OF:	Wake time	BREAKFAST		
		Fasting	After	Meds
MONDAY	a.m.			

Blood Pressure: ....

Pulse Rate:

TUESDAY	a.m.			

Blood Pressure: ....

Pulse Rate:

WEDNESDAY	a.m.			

Blood Pressure: ....

Pulse Rate:

THURSDAY	a.m.			

Blood Pressure: ....

Pulse Rate:

FRIDAY	a.m.			

Blood Pressure: ....

Pulse Rate:

SATURDAY	a.m.			

Blood Pressure: ....

Pulse Rate:

SUNDAY	a.m.			

Blood Pressure: ....

Pulse Rate:

My Blood Sugar Level

LUNCH			DINNER			Bedtime
Before	After	Meds	Before	After	Meds	
						p.m.

Notes: ....

						p.m.

Notes: ....

						p.m.

Notes: ....

						p.m.

Notes: ....

						p.m.

Notes: ....

						p.m.

Notes: ....

						p.m.

Notes: ....

Daily Tracking Log

WEEK OF:	Wake time	BREAKFAST		
		Fasting	After	Meds
MONDAY	a.m.			

Blood Pressure: ....

Pulse Rate:

TUESDAY	a.m.			

Blood Pressure: ....

Pulse Rate:

WEDNESDAY	a.m.			

Blood Pressure: ....

Pulse Rate:

THURSDAY	a.m.			

Blood Pressure: ....

Pulse Rate:

FRIDAY	a.m.			

Blood Pressure: ....

Pulse Rate:

SATURDAY	a.m.			

Blood Pressure: ....

Pulse Rate:

SUNDAY	a.m.			

Blood Pressure: ....

Pulse Rate:

My Blood Sugar Level

LUNCH			DINNER			Bedtime
Before	After	Meds	Before	After	Meds	
						p.m.

Notes: ....

						p.m.

Notes: ....

						p.m.

Notes: ....

						p.m.

Notes: ....

						p.m.

Notes: ....

						p.m.

Notes: ....

						p.m.

Notes: ....

Daily Tracking Log

WEEK OF:	Wake time	BREAKFAST		
		Fasting	After	Meds
MONDAY	a.m.			

Blood Pressure: ....

Pulse Rate:

TUESDAY	a.m.			

Blood Pressure: ....

Pulse Rate:

WEDNESDAY	a.m.			

Blood Pressure: ....

Pulse Rate:

THURSDAY	a.m.			

Blood Pressure: ....

Pulse Rate:

FRIDAY	a.m.			

Blood Pressure: ....

Pulse Rate:

SATURDAY	a.m.			

Blood Pressure: ....

Pulse Rate:

SUNDAY	a.m.			

Blood Pressure: ....

Pulse Rate:

My Blood Sugar Level

LUNCH			DINNER			Bedtime
Before	After	Meds	Before	After	Meds	
						p.m.

Notes: ....

						p.m.

Notes: ....

						p.m.

Notes: ....

						p.m.

Notes: ....

						p.m.

Notes: ....

						p.m.

Notes: ....

						p.m.

Notes: ....

Daily Tracking Log

WEEK OF:	Wake time	BREAKFAST		
		Fasting	After	Meds
MONDAY	a.m.			

Blood Pressure: ....

Pulse Rate:

TUESDAY	a.m.			

Blood Pressure: ....

Pulse Rate:

WEDNESDAY	a.m.			

Blood Pressure: ....

Pulse Rate:

THURSDAY	a.m.			

Blood Pressure: ....

Pulse Rate:

FRIDAY	a.m.			

Blood Pressure: ....

Pulse Rate:

SATURDAY	a.m.			

Blood Pressure: ....

Pulse Rate:

SUNDAY	a.m.			

Blood Pressure: ....

Pulse Rate:

My Blood Sugar Level

LUNCH			DINNER			Bedtime
Before	After	Meds	Before	After	Meds	
						p.m.

Notes: ....

						p.m.

Notes: ....

						p.m.

Notes: ....

						p.m.

Notes: ....

						p.m.

Notes: ....

						p.m.

Notes: ....

						p.m.

Notes: ....

Daily Tracking Log

WEEK OF:	Wake time	BREAKFAST		
		Fasting	After	Meds
MONDAY	a.m.			

Blood Pressure: ....

Pulse Rate:

TUESDAY	a.m.			

Blood Pressure: ....

Pulse Rate:

WEDNESDAY	a.m.			

Blood Pressure: ....

Pulse Rate:

THURSDAY	a.m.			

Blood Pressure: ....

Pulse Rate:

FRIDAY	a.m.			

Blood Pressure: ....

Pulse Rate:

SATURDAY	a.m.			

Blood Pressure: ....

Pulse Rate:

SUNDAY	a.m.			

Blood Pressure: ....

Pulse Rate:

My Blood Sugar Level

LUNCH			DINNER			Bedtime
Before	After	Meds	Before	After	Meds	
						p.m.

Notes: ....

						p.m.

Notes: ....

						p.m.

Notes: ....

						p.m.

Notes: ....

						p.m.

Notes: ....

						p.m.

Notes: ....

						p.m.

Notes: ....

Daily Tracking Log

WEEK OF:	Wake time	BREAKFAST		
		Fasting	After	Meds
MONDAY	a.m.			

Blood Pressure: ....

Pulse Rate:

TUESDAY	a.m.			

Blood Pressure: ....

Pulse Rate:

WEDNESDAY	a.m.			

Blood Pressure: ....

Pulse Rate:

THURSDAY	a.m.			

Blood Pressure: ....

Pulse Rate:

FRIDAY	a.m.			

Blood Pressure: ....

Pulse Rate:

SATURDAY	a.m.			

Blood Pressure: ....

Pulse Rate:

SUNDAY	a.m.			

Blood Pressure: ....

Pulse Rate:

My Blood Sugar Level

LUNCH			DINNER			Bedtime
Before	After	Meds	Before	After	Meds	
						p.m.

Notes: ....

						p.m.

Notes: ....

						p.m.

Notes: ....

						p.m.

Notes: ....

						p.m.

Notes: ....

						p.m.

Notes: ....

						p.m.

Notes: ....

Daily Tracking Log

WEEK OF:	Wake time	BREAKFAST		
		Fasting	After	Meds
MONDAY	a.m.			

Blood Pressure: ....

Pulse Rate:

TUESDAY	a.m.			

Blood Pressure: ....

Pulse Rate:

WEDNESDAY	a.m.			

Blood Pressure: ....

Pulse Rate:

THURSDAY	a.m.			

Blood Pressure: ....

Pulse Rate:

FRIDAY	a.m.			

Blood Pressure: ....

Pulse Rate:

SATURDAY	a.m.			

Blood Pressure: ....

Pulse Rate:

SUNDAY	a.m.			

Blood Pressure: ....

Pulse Rate:

My Blood Sugar Level

LUNCH			DINNER			Bedtime
Before	After	Meds	Before	After	Meds	
						p.m.

Notes: ....

						p.m.

Notes: ....

						p.m.

Notes: ....

						p.m.

Notes: ....

						p.m.

Notes: ....

						p.m.

Notes: ....

						p.m.

Notes: ....

Daily Tracking Log

WEEK OF:	Wake time	BREAKFAST		
		Fasting	After	Meds
MONDAY	a.m.			

Blood Pressure: ....

Pulse Rate:

TUESDAY	a.m.			

Blood Pressure: ....

Pulse Rate:

WEDNESDAY	a.m.			

Blood Pressure: ....

Pulse Rate:

THURSDAY	a.m.			

Blood Pressure: ....

Pulse Rate:

FRIDAY	a.m.			

Blood Pressure: ....

Pulse Rate:

SATURDAY	a.m.			

Blood Pressure: ....

Pulse Rate:

SUNDAY	a.m.			

Blood Pressure: ....

Pulse Rate:

My Blood Sugar Level

LUNCH			DINNER			Bedtime
Before	After	Meds	Before	After	Meds	
						p.m.

Notes: ....

						p.m.

Notes: ....

						p.m.

Notes: ....

						p.m.

Notes: ....

						p.m.

Notes: ....

						p.m.

Notes: ....

						p.m.

Notes: ....

Daily Tracking Log

WEEK OF:	Wake time	BREAKFAST		
		Fasting	After	Meds
MONDAY	a.m.			

Blood Pressure: ....

Pulse Rate:

TUESDAY	a.m.			

Blood Pressure: ....

Pulse Rate:

WEDNESDAY	a.m.			

Blood Pressure: ....

Pulse Rate:

THURSDAY	a.m.			

Blood Pressure: ....

Pulse Rate:

FRIDAY	a.m.			

Blood Pressure: ....

Pulse Rate:

SATURDAY	a.m.			

Blood Pressure: ....

Pulse Rate:

SUNDAY	a.m.			

Blood Pressure: ....

Pulse Rate:

My Blood Sugar Level

LUNCH			DINNER			Bedtime
Before	After	Meds	Before	After	Meds	
						p.m.

Notes: ....

						p.m.

Notes: ....

						p.m.

Notes: ....

						p.m.

Notes: ....

						p.m.

Notes: ....

						p.m.

Notes: ....

						p.m.

Notes: ....

Daily Tracking Log

WEEK OF:	Wake time	BREAKFAST		
		Fasting	After	Meds
MONDAY	a.m.			

Blood Pressure: ....

Pulse Rate:

TUESDAY	a.m.			

Blood Pressure: ....

Pulse Rate:

WEDNESDAY	a.m.			

Blood Pressure: ....

Pulse Rate:

THURSDAY	a.m.			

Blood Pressure: ....

Pulse Rate:

FRIDAY	a.m.			

Blood Pressure: ....

Pulse Rate:

SATURDAY	a.m.			

Blood Pressure: ....

Pulse Rate:

SUNDAY	a.m.			

Blood Pressure: ....

Pulse Rate:

My Blood Sugar Level

LUNCH			DINNER			Bedtime
Before	After	Meds	Before	After	Meds	
						p.m.

Notes: ....

						p.m.

Notes: ....

						p.m.

Notes: ....

						p.m.

Notes: ....

						p.m.

Notes: ....

						p.m.

Notes: ....

						p.m.

Notes: ....

Daily Tracking Log

WEEK OF:	Wake time	BREAKFAST		
		Fasting	After	Meds
MONDAY	a.m.			

Blood Pressure: ....

Pulse Rate:

TUESDAY	a.m.			

Blood Pressure: ....

Pulse Rate:

WEDNESDAY	a.m.			

Blood Pressure: ....

Pulse Rate:

THURSDAY	a.m.			

Blood Pressure: ....

Pulse Rate:

FRIDAY	a.m.			

Blood Pressure: ....

Pulse Rate:

SATURDAY	a.m.			

Blood Pressure: ....

Pulse Rate:

SUNDAY	a.m.			

Blood Pressure: ....

Pulse Rate:

My Blood Sugar Level

LUNCH			DINNER			Bedtime
Before	After	Meds	Before	After	Meds	
						p.m.

Notes: ....

						p.m.

Notes: ....

						p.m.

Notes: ....

						p.m.

Notes: ....

						p.m.

Notes: ....

						p.m.

Notes: ....

						p.m.

Notes: ....

Daily Tracking Log

WEEK OF:	Wake time	BREAKFAST		
		Fasting	After	Meds
MONDAY	a.m.			

Blood Pressure: ....

Pulse Rate:

TUESDAY	a.m.			

Blood Pressure: ....

Pulse Rate:

WEDNESDAY	a.m.			

Blood Pressure: ....

Pulse Rate:

THURSDAY	a.m.			

Blood Pressure: ....

Pulse Rate:

FRIDAY	a.m.			

Blood Pressure: ....

Pulse Rate:

SATURDAY	a.m.			

Blood Pressure: ....

Pulse Rate:

SUNDAY	a.m.			

Blood Pressure: ....

Pulse Rate:

My Blood Sugar Level

LUNCH			DINNER			Bedtime
Before	After	Meds	Before	After	Meds	
						p.m.

Notes: ....

						p.m.

Notes: ....

						p.m.

Notes: ....

						p.m.

Notes: ....

						p.m.

Notes: ....

						p.m.

Notes: ....

						p.m.

Notes: ....

Daily Tracking Log

WEEK OF:	Wake time	BREAKFAST		
		Fasting	After	Meds
MONDAY	a.m.			

Blood Pressure: ....

Pulse Rate:

TUESDAY	a.m.			

Blood Pressure: ....

Pulse Rate:

WEDNESDAY	a.m.			

Blood Pressure: ....

Pulse Rate:

THURSDAY	a.m.			

Blood Pressure: ....

Pulse Rate:

FRIDAY	a.m.			

Blood Pressure: ....

Pulse Rate:

SATURDAY	a.m.			

Blood Pressure: ....

Pulse Rate:

SUNDAY	a.m.			

Blood Pressure: ....

Pulse Rate:

My Blood Sugar Level

LUNCH			DINNER			Bedtime
Before	After	Meds	Before	After	Meds	
						p.m.

Notes: ....

| | | | | | | p.m. |

Notes: ....

| | | | | | | p.m. |

Notes: ....

| | | | | | | p.m. |

Notes: ....

| | | | | | | p.m. |

Notes: ....

| | | | | | | p.m. |

Notes: ....

| | | | | | | p.m. |

Notes: ....

Daily Tracking Log

WEEK OF:	Wake time	BREAKFAST		
		Fasting	After	Meds
MONDAY	a.m.			

Blood Pressure: ....

Pulse Rate:

TUESDAY	a.m.			

Blood Pressure: ....

Pulse Rate:

WEDNESDAY	a.m.			

Blood Pressure: ....

Pulse Rate:

THURSDAY	a.m.			

Blood Pressure: ....

Pulse Rate:

FRIDAY	a.m.			

Blood Pressure: ....

Pulse Rate:

SATURDAY	a.m.			

Blood Pressure: ....

Pulse Rate:

SUNDAY	a.m.			

Blood Pressure: ....

Pulse Rate:

My Blood Sugar Level

LUNCH			DINNER			Bedtime
Before	After	Meds	Before	After	Meds	
						p.m.

Notes: ....

						p.m.

Notes: ....

						p.m.

Notes: ....

						p.m.

Notes: ....

						p.m.

Notes: ....

						p.m.

Notes: ....

						p.m.

Notes: ....

Daily Tracking Log

WEEK OF:	Wake time	BREAKFAST		
		Fasting	After	Meds
MONDAY	a.m.			

Blood Pressure: ....

Pulse Rate:

TUESDAY	a.m.			

Blood Pressure: ....

Pulse Rate:

WEDNESDAY	a.m.			

Blood Pressure: ....

Pulse Rate:

THURSDAY	a.m.			

Blood Pressure: ....

Pulse Rate:

FRIDAY	a.m.			

Blood Pressure: ....

Pulse Rate:

SATURDAY	a.m.			

Blood Pressure: ....

Pulse Rate:

SUNDAY	a.m.			

Blood Pressure: ....

Pulse Rate:

My Blood Sugar Level

| LUNCH | | | DINNER | | | Bedtime |
Before	After	Meds	Before	After	Meds	
						p.m.

Notes: ....

						p.m.

Notes: ....

						p.m.

Notes: ....

						p.m.

Notes: ....

						p.m.

Notes: ....

						p.m.

Notes: ....

						p.m.

Notes: ....

Daily Tracking Log

WEEK OF:	Wake time	BREAKFAST		
		Fasting	After	Meds
MONDAY	a.m.			

Blood Pressure: ....

Pulse Rate:

TUESDAY	a.m.			

Blood Pressure: ....

Pulse Rate:

WEDNESDAY	a.m.			

Blood Pressure: ....

Pulse Rate:

THURSDAY	a.m.			

Blood Pressure: ....

Pulse Rate:

FRIDAY	a.m.			

Blood Pressure: ....

Pulse Rate:

SATURDAY	a.m.			

Blood Pressure: ....

Pulse Rate:

SUNDAY	a.m.			

Blood Pressure: ....

Pulse Rate:

My Blood Sugar Level

LUNCH			DINNER			Bedtime
Before	After	Meds	Before	After	Meds	
						p.m.

Notes: ....

						p.m.

Notes: ....

						p.m.

Notes: ....

						p.m.

Notes: ....

						p.m.

Notes: ....

						p.m.

Notes: ....

						p.m.

Notes: ....

Daily Tracking Log

WEEK OF:	Wake time	BREAKFAST		
		Fasting	After	Meds
MONDAY	a.m.			

Blood Pressure: ....

Pulse Rate:

TUESDAY	a.m.			

Blood Pressure: ....

Pulse Rate:

WEDNESDAY	a.m.			

Blood Pressure: ....

Pulse Rate:

THURSDAY	a.m.			

Blood Pressure: ....

Pulse Rate:

FRIDAY	a.m.			

Blood Pressure: ....

Pulse Rate:

SATURDAY	a.m.			

Blood Pressure: ....

Pulse Rate:

SUNDAY	a.m.			

Blood Pressure: ....

Pulse Rate:

My Blood Sugar Level

LUNCH			DINNER			Bedtime
Before	After	Meds	Before	After	Meds	
						p.m.

Notes: ....

						p.m.

Notes: ....

						p.m.

Notes: ....

						p.m.

Notes: ....

						p.m.

Notes: ....

						p.m.

Notes: ....

						p.m.

Notes: ....

Made in the USA
Monee, IL
07 October 2023